Table of Contents

Diverticulosis and diverticulitis are two conditions that occur in your large intestine (colon). Together they are known as diverticular disease. Both share the common feature of diverticula. Diverticula are one or more pockets or bulges that form in the wall of your colon.

Diverticula are like expanded areas or bubbles that form when you fill the inner tube of a bike tire with too much air. The increase in pressure from too much air being pumped into the inner tube causes the bubble to form where the rubber is the weakest. Similarly, an increase in pressure inside the colon causes pockets or bulges (diverticula) to form in weakened areas of your colon's walls.

Diverticula can range from pea-size to much larger. Although they can form anywhere in the inner lining of your colon, they are most commonly found in your lower left side, in the S-shaped segment of your colon called the sigmoid colon.

BREAKFAST

1. Creamy, Dairy-Free Pumpkin Alfredo

Prep Time: 35 Minutes

Cook Time: 50 Minutes

Servings: 4

Ingredients

- 250g Pasta (we used GF brown rice fettuccini)
- 2 tbsp Olive Oil
- 2 tbsp minced Garlic
- 1.5 cups Unsweetened Almond Milk, divided
- 1/2 cup Pumpkin Puree (NOT pumpkin pie filling)
- Salt & pepper to taste
- 1 tbsp Cornstarch
- 1 tbsp Lemon Juice
- 1/4 cup Nutritional Yeast
- Fresh Oregano or Basil for garnish *optional*
- Stove top frying pan
- Large Pot

Instructions

Cook your pasta accordingly.

1. While your pasta is cooking, heat your olive oil in a frying pan to a medium-high heat. Add in garlic and cook until it begins to brown. Add in 1 cup of almond milk (reserve the other 1/2 cup), pumpkin puree, salt & pepper and cook for a few minutes.
2. In a separate bowl, mix the tablespoon of cornstarch with the other half cup of almond milk until the cornstarch is dissolved. Add the mixture to the pan, as well as the lemon juice & nutritional yeast.
3. Continue to cook until the sauce thickens, then add it to your cooked & strained pasta and toss to coat.
4. Garnish with additional salt and pepper, along with some fresh herbs such as oregano or basil, if you wish!

Prep Time: 50 Minutes

Cook Time: 35 Minutes

Servings: 12

Ingredients

- 1 8oz block Cream Cheese, room temperature
- 1 8oz container Vegetable or Herb Cream Cheese
- 2 tbsp Powdered Ranch Seasoning
- 1/4 cup Green Onions, chopped
- 1/4 cup Red Pepper (keep that green stem!)
- 2 cups Cheddar Cheese, shredded (1 cup for inside the cheese ball, 1 cup to coat it)
- Mixer
- Mixing Bowl
- Plastic Wrap
- 4 Rubber Bands/Elastics

Instructions

1. In a mixing bowl, combine your cream cheeses until smooth. Stir in the ranch seasoning, green onions, red pepper and 1 cup of cheddar cheese.

2. Lay out plastic wrap, and in the centre place some of the cheddar cheese shredding. Scoop the cheese ball mixture into the centre and begin creating your ball form coating with the rest of the cheddar cheese on all sides.

3. Once you're happy with how coated the ball is in shredded cheddar, wrap it up completely with your plastic wrap, and continue to shape it into a ball form. Then, wrap it again with a second layer of plastic wrap to ensure it's contained well, and held in tightly.

4. Next, place 4 elastics around the ball to create a pumpkin shape. Refridgerate for 2-3 hours or overnight. Double up the elastics if you need them to be tighter to create the form you'd like.

5. Remove from fridge, and cut off the elastics and remove the plastic wrap. Place it in the centre of your serving platter, and surround with serving crackers. Place the stem top from your red pepper in the centre of the cheese ball, and serve immediately!

Prep Time: 10 Minutes

Cook Time: 30 Minutes

Servings: 4

Ingredients

- 1 butternut squash
- 2 tbsps olive oil
- 1 1/2 lbs mild Italian turkey sausage, casings removed
- 1 onion, chopped
- 1 package (or 8oz) baby kale, pre-chopped or fresh, stems removed
- 1 tbsp minced garlic
- 1/2 cup chicken broth
- 1 tsp red wine vinegar (can substitute for apple cider vinegar)
- 1/4 tsp red pepper flakes
- 2 tsp rosemary
- 2 tsp fresh sage, chopped
- salt & pepper, to taste
- Baking sheet
- Large non-stick baking pan

Instructions

1. Preheat oven to 425 degrees.

2. Next, cut the bulb end off of your butternut squash, as well as the top stem creating two flat ends. Peel the squash, and place in your stand spiralizer and spiralize into noodles.

3. Toss the butternut squash noodles in 1 tbsp of olive oil, and sprinkle with salt & pepper. Spread them out on an even layer on a non-stick baking sheet (or one lined with parchment paper) and bake for 15 minutes. Toss, then continue baking for an additional 15 minutes, or until lightly browned, and tender.

4. While the squash noodles are baking, heat your non-stick baking pan to a medium heat. Add 1 tbsp olive oil, and brown and crumble the turkey sausage until fully cooked, and sprinkle with a bit of salt & pepper. If you bought sausages in casings, make sure you squeeze the meat from the casings before this.

5. Add in your chopped onion, and cook with the sausage for another 3-4 minutes or until translucent and softened.

6. Next, add the kale and stir until it's wilted (don't worry if it seems like a lot in the pan, it will shrink down significantly!).

7. Add the minced garlic, chicken stock, vinegar, pepper flakes, rosemary and sage. Mix well, and continue cooking for an additional few minutes. Make sure you do this uncovered, as it will reduce the liquid as it cooks.

8. Add your cooked butternut squash noodles (now removed from the oven) and toss. The noodles will break up as you toss them, and that's okay...just means that they are so tender and delicious!

9. Ready to serve!

Prep Time: 40 Minutes

Cook Time: 55 Minutes

Servings: 6-8

Ingredients

- 1/4 cup olive oil
- 2 tbsp red wine vinegar
- 1 tbsp balsamic vinegar
- 1/2 lemon, juiced
- 1/2 tsp dried oregano
- 1 tsp dried basil
- 2 tsp minced garlic
- ½ tsp each salt and pepper
- 4-5 cups cooked chilled quinoa
- 1.5 cups cherry tomatoes, halved
- 1 cucumber, diced
- 1 yellow pepper, diced
- 1/2 cup kalamata olives, sliced
- 1/2 red onion, finely chopped
- 2/3 cup feta cheese, crumbled

Instructions

1. Add olive oil, vinegars, lemon juice, oregano, basil, garlic, salt, and pepper to a jar or container. Lid the jar and shake thoroughly to combine. Set aside.
2. In a large bowl, combine remaining ingredients and mix gently.
3. Just before serving, give the dressing another quick shake and pour over the salad. Mix gently to coat all ingredients. Serve immediately.

Prep Time: 10 Minutes

Cook Time: 35-40 Minutes

Servings: 4

Ingredients

- 1 large sweet potato, peeled & diced into cubes
- 4 tbsp olive oil
- 1 lb chicken breast, diced into cubes
- 1/2 pkg of extra firm tofu, pressed and cubed
- 4 cups baby Brussels sprouts
- 1/2 red onion, diced into large chunks
- 4 cloves of garlic, minced
- 1 tsp dried sage
- 1 tsp dried parsley
- 1 tsp dried rosemary
- Pinch of nutmeg
- Salt & pepper, to taste
- 1/2 cup pecans
- 1/3 cup dried cranberries
- Sheet Pan
- Aluminum Foil

Instructions

1. Preheat oven to 400 degrees Fahrenheit.

2. Line your sheet pan with foil, drizzle half your olive oil and place sweet potatoes onto the pan with some salt & pepper. Toss until coated and roast for 15 minutes.

3. Remove sweet potatoes from the oven, and carefully make a small dividing wall in the centre of the pan with the foil. Divide all your veggies between both halves. Next, add your tofu to one half, and your chicken to the other. Drizzle with the rest of the olive oil, and add in all your seasonings. Toss, and bake for 20 minutes (or until chicken is completely cooked through).

4. Once removed from the oven, add in pecan & dried cranberries. Serve immediately!

Prep Time: 25 Minutes

Cook Time: 40 Minutes

Servings: 4

Ingredients

- 1 1/2 cup raw cashews, soaked
- 3 tbsp nutritional yeast
- 1 tsp salt
- 1 tsp garlic, minced
- 1/2 tsp chili powder
- 6 pickled jalapeño slices
- 6-8 tbsp pickled jalapeño juice
- Hot water
- 2 bags vegan corn tortilla chips
- 1/2 cup black beans
- 1/4 cup green onions
- 1/2 cup tomatoes, diced
- Jalapeño slices (as many as you want)
- Sheet Pan

Instructions

1. Preheat oven to 350 degrees Fahrenheit.

2. Quick soak cashews by placing them in very hot water for roughly 30-60 minutes.

3. In a food processor, combine soaked cashews, nutritional yeast, salt, chili powder, jalapeño slices, and jalapeño juice. Blend until smooth.

4. If the sauce is too thick for drizzling, add hot water or more jalapeño juice a little bit at a time to thin.

5. Arrange tortilla chips on a baking tray. Top with beans, tomatoes, green onions, and jalapeño slices. Drizzle generously with queso sauce.

6. Bake for 10 minutes or until heated through. Serve hot!

Prep Time: 10 Minutes

Cook Time: 30-45 Minutes

Servings: 4

Ingredients

- 1 medium sweet potato, peeled and chopped
- 1-2 cups green beans
- 2 cups Brussels sprouts, halved
- 2 bell peppers, chopped
- 4 turkey sausages, cut into 1 inch pieces
- 1/2 tsp garlic powder
- 1 tbsp dried oregano
- 1 tbsp dried parsley
- 1 tbsp dried rosemary
- 1 tsp paprika
- 6 tbsp olive oil
- 1/2 teaspoon red chili flakes
- S&P, to taste (pinch of each)
- Baking Sheet/Pan

- Parchment paper or non-stick foil (if not using a non-stick pan)

Instructions

1. Preheat oven to 400 degrees F.
2. Line your baking sheet, if needed.
3. Prep your vegetables, and cut up your sausage.
4. Add olive oil, and spices/seasonings and mix until well coated.
5. Place all the vegetables and sausage onto your baking sheet, and spread out evening to cook.
6. Cook for 15-20 minutes, then gently mix/flip/stir everything around to bake evenly. Return to the oven for an additional 15-20 minutes or until the sausage is cooked through, and the veggies are tender and crisp on the edges.
7. Serve over quinoa or rice, and optionally top with parmesan cheese.

Prep Time: 5 Minutes

Cook Time: 25-30 Minutes

Servings: 2-3

Ingredients

- 1 large sweet potato, cubed
- 1/2 large red onion, wedge sliced
- 2 zucchini diced
- 1 can kernel corn, drained
- 1 can chickpeas, drained & rinsed
- Olive Oil
- Salt & Pepper

Moroccan Seasoning:

- 1 tsp of each - cumin, chili powder, garlic powder, turmeric and 1/4 tsp of salt & pepper)
- Avocado halves, sliced & fanned
- 4 cups cooked brown rice (sub for quinoa, white rice, or lettuce)

Tahini Sauce:

- 1/4 cup tahini, 1 tbsp maple syrup, tbsp lemon juice, 2-4 tbsp hot water to thin
- Sheet Pan
- Bowls for serving

Instructions

1. Preheat your oven to 400 degrees Fahrenheit.
2. Place your diced sweet potatoes in the microwave for 2 minutes to soften before roasting.
3. On your sheet pan, lay out the sweet potatoes, onion, corn, zucchini and chickpeas in rows.
4. Drizzle the whole pan with olive oil, and sprinkle the veggies with salt & pepper, leaving chickpeas alone. Toss the veggies individually to coat.
5. Mix up your Moroccan seasoning, and sprinkle over the chickpeas, tossing to coat.
6. Bake for 25-30 minutes or until veggies are roasted to your liking.
7. While the sheet pan bakes, mix up your tahini sauce.
8. Remove sheet pan from oven, and spoon the chickpeas & veggies into your bowl with your rice at the bottom.

9. Top with avocado & drizzle with tahini sauce before
    enjoying!

Prep Time: 5 Minutes

Cook Time: 25-30 Minutes

Servings: 10

Ingredients

- 1 pound ground beef
- 1 tbsp minced garlic
- ¼ cup onion, diced
- 1 tsp salt
- 4 slices American Cheese
- 10 dill pickle slices
- 10 mini slider buns
- Lettuce
- 1-2 tbsp olive oil
- Kabob skewers
- Frying pan

Instructions

1. Cut each cheese slice into four squares. Cut lettuce into large pieces. Slice pickles if they are not pre-sliced.

2. In a bowl, mix beef, minced garlic, onion, and salt. Pinch off a piece of the mixture and roll into a ball. Place in the palm of your hand and press down slightly to flatten the patty until it's about 1 inch thick. Repeat for all of the meat.

3. Heat oil in a large frying pan on medium-high heat.

4. Cook mini patties in a frying pan for about 1-2 minutes per side until the internal temperature reaches 160°F. Repeat for all patties. As patties come out, place a piece of cheese on top, allowing to melt slightly.

5. Build the skewers by spreading Big Mac sauce on the bottom bun, then sliding on the bottom half of the bun, burger patty, cheese slice, folded up lettuce square, pickle slice, more Big Mac Sauce and top bun.

6. Serve skewers with the extra Copycat Big Mac Sauce on the side for dipping, if desired. Enjoy!

Servings: 4-6

Ingredients

- 1 medium to large butternut squash, halved, pelled and seeded
- 2 tbsp butter, melted (we used a vegan variety)
- 2 tbsp olive oil
- 4 tbsp garlic, minced
- Salt & pepper, to taste
- 1 tsp cajun seasoning
- Fresh Thyme (about 2 long sprigs cut up)
- Casserole Dish or Roasting Pan
- Sharp Knife
- Spoon
- Peeler

Instructions

1. Preheat oven to 425 degrees Fahrenheit.

2. Cut your butternut squash in half lengthwise, remove the seeds with a spoon, and use a peeler to remove all the skin.

3. Brush with olive oil and sprinkle with salt and pepper, and roast with the cut sides facing down for 20 minutes or until softened.

4. Remove from oven, and carefully remove from your roasting dish onto a cutting board. With a sharp knife beging to cut slits down the back of the squash about 3/4 of the way through in thin slices. Go slow if needed to be sure you're not cutting through the squash.

5. Return to the roasting dish, and mix your melted butter, cajun seasoning and garlic and begin brushing it over the now sliced backs of the squash. Sprinkle salt & pepper on top, and place some sprigs of fresh thyme as well.

6. Return to the oven and roast for an additional 30 or more minutes, basting with the juices every 10 minutes.

7. Once browned and fully cooked to your liking (this will greatly depend on the size of your squash) then remove from the oven, baste and top with more fresh thyme. You can serve right out of the dish

immediately or place onto a serving platter. Add more salt & pepper if desired.

11. Bloody Mary Sheet Pan Chicken

Prep Time: 30 Minutes

Cook Time: 20 Minutes

Servings: 4-6

Ingredients

- 4 chicken breasts, cubed
- 1 medium red onion, diced
- 1 cup grape tomatoes, halved
- 1 cup chopped celery
- 1 can tomato juice (we used V8 Seasoned)
- 2 tbsp minced garlic, divided
- 1 tbsp worcestershire sauce
- 1 tsp hot sauce
- 2 tbsps celery salt, divided
- 1 tbsp olive oil
- 1 lime, for squeezing
- Cooked pasta & vodka sauce for serving, optional
- Bacon bits, optional for garnish.
- Sheet Pan

- Parchment Paper (optional)

Instructions

1. Preheat oven to 375 degrees Fahrenheit.

2. Place your chopped chicken breast into a medium sized mixing bowl and add the following for it's marinade: tomato juice, 1 tbsp minced garlic, worcestershire sauce, hot sauce, 1 tbsp celery salt. Set aside.

3. Next, add your chopped onion, tomatoes and celery to your parchment-lined sheet pan, and drizzle with olive oil, adding 1 tbsp minced garlic and 1 tbsp celery salt, toss to coat.

4. Moving the vegetables to the top and bottom of your sheet pan, add your marinated chicken to the sheet pan and spread out evenly.

5. Cook in the oven for 20 minutes, turning/tossing half way through. Remove when chicken is fully cooked. Drizzle with freshly squeezed lime juice.

6. Serve immediately over pasta in vodka sauce, on it's own, on rice or enjoy on it's own! Optionally, top with some bacon bits for some added smokiness to your meal. Enjoy!

12. Simple Salmon Sheet Pan

Prep Time: 15 Minutes

Cook Time: 45 Minutes

Servings: 6

Ingredients

- 1 whole, skin-on salmon fillet
- 1 1/2 cups mini potatoes, quartered
- 2 cups green beans, ends snipped
- 3-4 tbsps olive oil
- 1/4 cup honey
- 1/4 cup grainy dijon mustard
- 1 tbsp garlic, minced
- 1 tsp ginger, minced
- 1 pinch red pepper flakes
- 1 tsp fresh thyme, chopped
- 1/2 lemon, juiced
- Parsley, chopped
- Salt & pepper
- Sheet Pan

Instructions

1. Preheat oven to 400 Degrees Fahrenheit.
2. Place the salmon fillet, mini potatoes, and green beans onto the sheet pan. Drizzle with olive oil and season with salt and pepper. Toss to coat.
3. In a small bowl, combine honey, dijon, garlic, ginger, red pepper flakes, and thyme. Mix well. Reserve 1/4 cup of the marinade.
4. Pour remaining marinade onto salmon and spread evenly with a fork or spoon to coat.
5. Bake in oven for 20-25 minutes.
6. Remove from oven and spread the reserved marinade onto the salmon fillet.
7. Return to the oven and Broil on High for 3-5 minutes.
8. When fully cooked, remove from oven. Top with freshly squeezed lemon juice and fresh parsley.
9. Serve warm and enjoy!

Prep Time: 10 mins

Cook Time: 30 mins

Servings: 4

Ingredients

- 4 chicken breasts (approx 1.25lbs)
- 2/3 cup balsamic vinegar
- 2/3 cup fat free Italian salad dressing
- 1 head of broccoli, stalks removed and chopped
- 1 cup baby carrots
- 2 cups Brussels sprouts, halved
- 1/2 pint cherry tomatoes
- 2 tsp Italian seasoning
- 3 tbsp olive oil
- 1 tbsp minced garlic
- salt & pepper
- Mixing Bowl
- Non-Stick Baking Sheet (or parchment lined)

Instructions

1. Preheat your oven to 400 degrees F. If not using a non stick pan, line with non-stick foil or parchment paper.

2. In a large mixing bowl, combine the balsamic vinegar and Italian dressing (we used a fat-free variety, but use whatever you have on hand).

3. Add your chicken and veggies to the mix and toss until everything is well coated in the marinade. Optionally, you can set aside for 30 minutes to give it more flavor, but if you're short on time, don't worry about it!

4. Place the chicken on the pan first, then surround it with the vegetables and drizzle any extra marinade over everything.

5. Roast in your pre-heated oven for 20-30 minutes. Double check to make sure the chicken breast is fully cooked, if not, continue roasting for 5 minutes at a time.

6. Serve over rice or quinoa, or on it's own!

Prep Time: 30 Minutes

Cook Time: 30 Minutes

Servings: 4

Ingredients

Salad Bowls:

- 4 cups shredded napa or green cabbage
- 2 tablespoons chopped fresh mint
- 2 tablespoons chopped fresh basil
- 2 cups cooked bulgur
- 1 red bell pepper, chopped
- 4 medium carrots, peeled and chopped
- 1 yellow bell pepper, chopped
- 1 medium cucumber, chopped
- 1 cup canned whole beets, chopped
- 2 tablespoons sesame seeds

Peanut Sauce

- ½ cup smooth natural peanut butter
- ¼ cup reduced-sodium soy sauce
- ¼ cup water

- 1 tablespoon rice vinegar
- 1 tablespoon honey
- 1 clove garlic, minced

Instructions

1. Combine cabbage, mint and basil in a large bowl. Divide the mixture among 4 single-serving lidded containers. Top each with 1/2 cup cooked bulgur and equal parts of red bell pepper, carrots, yellow bell pepper, cucumber, beets and sesame seeds.
2. Whisk peanut butter, soy sauce, water, vinegar, honey and garlic in a small bowl. Divide the peanut sauce among 4 small lidded containers and refrigerate.
3. Seal the salad containers and refrigerate for up to 4 days. Dress with peanut sauce just before serving.

Prep Time: 40 Minutes

Cook Time: 35 Minutes

Servings: 3

Ingredients

- 100 grams white basmati rice
- 6 green beans
- 1/2 cup diced, roasted red pepper (peeled)
- 1/4 ripe avocado (sliced lengthways)
- 1/2 cup Lebanese cucumber (very finely sliced)
- 6 stems tinned asparagus
- 1 tin tuna slices (VG and vegetarian swap with thin slices of flavoured tofu)
- 1/2 cup pumpkin chunks (peeled and roasted)
- 1/2 lemon (cut into quarters)
- 2 teaspoons pickled ginger

Dressing:

- 1/2 cup freshly squeezed orange juice
- 4 tablespoons sesame oil
- pinch of salt and pepper to taste

Instructions

1. Cook rice and drain
   Blanche green beans
   Grill red pepper and remove skin and dice
   Thinly slice avocado lengthways
   Slice cucumber thinly
   Drain 6 stems of asparagus
   Drain tuna slices of oil
   Boil pumpkin chunks until tender but firm enough to place on a place

2. Decoration:
   Place the red pepper in a mound in the middle of both plates/bowls
   Arrange the other ingredients from middle to outer edge in a clocklike arrangement on both plates/bowls, spreading the ingredients out so there are no gaps at the edges of the bowl

3. Dressing:

   Shake OJ and sesame oil vigorously add salt and pepper to taste
   Pour dressing over the bowl and place pickle ginger

slices on green beans and lemon slice on the avocado
for a colour contrast

Prep Time: 30 Minutes

Cook Time:55 Minutes

Servings: 2

Ingredients

- 225 grams pizza sauce (garlic, onion and herb flavour)
- 20 ml extra-virgin olive oil
- extra-virgin olive oil spray
- plain greek yoghurt
- juice of one whole lime
- 1 teaspoon onion powder
- 1 teaspoon garlic powder
- 1/2 teaspoon sweet paprika
- 250 grams 25% reduced fat mature cheddar cheese
- 250 grams cooked shredded chicken (or 1 cup plain firm tofu for vegetarians)
- 400 grams white potato (skinned peeled)
- 400 grams basmati rice (cooked and drained)
- salt and pepper to taste
- 6 large flour tortillas

Instructions

1. Heat oven to 210C

2. Spray potatoes with olive oil spray and mix sweet paprika powder through and bake for 20 minutes or until the potatoes are soft on inside and crispy on the outside

3. Put olive oil garlic and onion powder into a frypan and gently heat for one minute.

4. Add chicken (or firm tofu) and 180 grams of pizza sauce, coat and mix in chicken (or tofu) and add lime juice and salt and pepper to taste.

5. Lay out tortillas on a clean dry surface, divide baked potato, rice, chicken mixture (or tofu) into six and layer them in the centre of each tortilla, top with cheese leaving ¼ cup for decoration.

6. Tuck the ends of the tortillas inward over the mixture and roll the burritos tightly and place lip side down in a deep dish

7. Paint the tops of the tortillas with the remaining pizza sauce and sprinkle remaining cheese on top and cover and bake for 15-20 minutes

8. Serve with a dollop of plain yoghurt on top

Prep Time: 35 Minutes

Cook Time: 45 Minutes

Servings: 4

Ingredients

- olive oil spray
- 1/2 cup cranberry jelly
- 400 grams brie cheese
- 1/2 cup white breadcrumbs
- 2 kg (large) turkey breast fillet
- 1 cup low salt chicken stock
- 1 cup white wine
- pinch of all spice
- 2 tablespoons pure honey
- kitchen string
- wire baking rack

Instructions

1. Preheat oven to 200C
   Place turkey breast on a clean kitchen board and slice

sideways through the breast don't cut all the way through as you are going to open the breast out and lie it flat on the board

Turn the breast over and spread jam down the middle

Thinly slice brie cheese and lay on top of the jam down the middle, top with breadcrumbs

Fold the sides in to wrap the stuffing inside the breast

Scure the roll with kitchen string at 3-4cm intervals to bind the roll tightly enclosing the cheese and walnut inside the roll

Place the roll on a wire baking rack in a roasting pan

Spray the top of the roll with olive oil and season with salt and pepper

Pour stock, wine and spoon honey into the bottom of the baking tin add pinch of all spice

Roast the turkey for 50-70 minutes, basting every 8-10 minutes with the liquid in the tray until when you piece the roll the juice is clear

Take the roll out and wrap in foil and set aside for 15 minutes

Pour the juice into a saucepan and boil vigorously to reduce volume

Unwrap, slice the roll on a service dish and gently remove kitchen string

Pour the reduced juice over the turkey
Serve with your favourite salad or vegetables

Prep Time: 45 Minutes

Cook Time: 55 Minutes

Servings: 3

Ingredients

- 280 grams firm tofu cut into small bite sized blocks
- 100 grams dry penne pasta
- 300 ml passata
- 1 small red onion blended and press the juice out (do not use the pulp)
- 2 teaspoons garlic powder
- 1 lemon juiced
- 2 tablespoons soy sauce
- 1 cup milk of your choice
- 1/4 cup water
- 1 teaspoon smoky paprika
- 6 tablespoons nutritional yeast
- 1 red capsicum diced
- 1 tablespoon flour of your choice
- 100 grams yoghurt of your choice (to serve)
- 1 tablespoon powdered oregano

- 50 grams corn kernels
- 3 grinds of black pepper

Instructions

2. Place the tofu in a bowl and marinate in thoroughly mixed, lemon juice, paprika and soy mixture for at least 30 minutes for a full flavour.
3. Place milk, garlic, black pepper, oregano, nutritional yeast and tomatoes into a blender and process.
4. Cook pasta until al dente, in the meantime cook the tofu in olive oil until it is golden on each side, set aside.
5. In a heavy pan cook the onion and red pepper in water for 3-5 minutes until tender, then add the tomato mix into the pan, gently stir in the flour and simmer until the sauce thickens.
6. Mix the tofu, pasta and sauce together and top with the yoghurt.

19. Beetroot Carrot Salad

Prep Time: 45 Minutes

Cook Time: 55 Minutes

Servings: 3

Ingredients

- 3 golden beetroots (peeled) or 3 large carrots (skin left on) or mixture of both
- 500 grams haloumi (thickly sliced)
- 1 teaspoon fresh oregano leaves
- 100 ml maple syrup
- 50 ml fresh lemon juice
- 50 grams spinach leaves
- 200 grams hulled tahini
- 100 grams noodles
- 2 tablespoons extra virgin olive oil

Instructions

1. Preheat the oven for 10 minutes at 180C. Wrap the beetroot and/or carrots in foil and place in the oven

for 40 minutes or until cooked through. Put aside to cool then cut into wedges.

2. In a saucepan, heat olive oil to a medium heat and brown the haloumi on both sides.

3. Turn the heat down and add the maple syrup, lemon juice and oregano and stir through.

4. Place a tablespoon of hulled tahini on each serving plate and a few baby spinach leaves on top, then add the haloumi and the beetroot/carrot wedges.

5. Sprinkle with crispy noodles and top with left over juice.

Prep Time: 45 Minutes

Cook Time: 55 Minutes

Servings: 3

Ingredients

- 8 lean chicken sausages
- 1 red apple (peeled, cored and cut into thick wedges)
- 2 medium peeled carrots
- 50 grams chopped yellow squash
- 1 teaspoon garlic powder
- 1 tablespoon dried italian herbs
- 1 tablespoon extra-virgin olive oil
- 400 ml a dry cider
- 200 ml low sodium chicken or vegetable stock
- 1 tablespoon arrowroot flour
- 50 ml pouring cream

Instruction

1. Heat oil in a thick bottomed pan and gently fry the sausages until golden brown

2. Take the sausages out and put them aside

3. Put the pan back on medium heat and add apple squash and carrot, and cook until soft

4. Add cider, stock, herbs, garlic powder and sift in flour and stir until thickened a little

5. Add the sausages and simmer for 5-10 minutes

6. Add cream and simmer for a further 5-10 minutes, add more flour if you want a thicker sauce

21. Dijon Tofu Ciabatta

Prep Time: 10 minutes

Cook Time: 35 minutes

Serving: 4

Ingredients

- 400 grams tofu cut into 100 grams slabs
- 1/2 ripe avocado peeled and mashed
- 50 grams baby spinach leaves
- 4 slices tasty cheddar
- 30 ml lemon juice
- 30 grams whole egg mayonnaise
- 30 grams Dijon mustard
- 1 tablespoon soy sauce
- 50 ml Extra virgin olive oil
- 1 teaspoon smoky paprika
- Salt and pepper to taste
- 4 crusty white ciabatta rolls (gluten free roll if desired)
- 1 zip lock bag to marinate the tofu in

Instructions

1. Season the tofu with salt and pepper – rub it in
2. Add 50 ml of olive oil, smokey paprika, lemon juice, and soy sauce into a ziplocked bag, add the tofu and coat with the marinade, leave in the fridge of 2 hours.
3. Warm the BBQ to medium heat.
4. Add 30 grams of Dijon mustard to whole egg mayonnaise and blend thoroughly.
5. Take the tofu out of the fridge and out of the bag, grill each side of 2-3 minutes until golden.
6. Spread one side of each roll with Dijon/mayonnaise mix and the other side with mashed avocado.
7. Place a slice of cheese on the mayonnaise side and baby spinach leaves on the avocado side, press down slightly so they are a little embedded in the avocado (makes it easier to close the roll).
8. Slice the tofu in thin strips and pile them evenly on the rocket side of each roll and close the roll.
9. Serve immediately.

Prep Time: 10 minutes

Cook Time: 30-40 minutes

Servings: 4

Ingredients

- 4 boneless skinless chicken breasts
- 4 slices of provolone cheese, halved
- 8 dill pickle slices
- 1 egg, beaten
- 1 cup panko breadcrumbs (we used gluten free)
- 1/2 cup fresh dill, chopped
- 3 cups mini potatoes
- 2 cups rainbow carrots (or mini carrots)
- 1 tbsp olive oil
- 1 tbsp garlic
- 1/2 lemon, juiced
- Salt & Pepper, to taste
- 1/4 cup light mayo
- 1/4 cup light sour cream
- tbsp lemon juice
- tbsp fresh dill

- Sharp Knife
- Sheet Pan
- Pastry Brush
- Small mixing bowl

Instructions

1. Preheat your own to 400 degrees Fahrenheit.

2. Using a sharp knife, slice your chicken breasts in half, lengthwise, but not all the way through. This creates a pocket that you can now add 2 pickle slices and 2 halves of provolone cheese to the center of each chicken breast.

3. On your sheet pan, place your mini potatoes and carrots, and drizzle with olive oil, minced garlic, some of your of freshly chopped dill and lemon juice. Mix well with your hands so all the veggies are well coated. Push the veggies to the edges of the pan, place your 4 stuffed chicken breasts onto the pan. Fill in any gaps with the carrots and potatoes so the pan is nice and full, and can cook evenly.

4. Next, brush the tops of each chicken breast with your egg wash. Top with a mixture of panko breadcrumbs

and some more freshly chopped dill. Sprinkle salt and pepper over the entire pan.

5. Bake for 30-40 minutes, depending on the size of your chicken breasts, or until everything is fully cooked through.

6. While everything is baking, in a small bowl, mix together your mayo, sour cream, lemon juice and fresh dill to make a dill serving sauce (this is optional, of course!).

7. Remove your chicken and veggies from the oven, and serve, topped with your dill sauce.

Prep Time: 30 Minutes

Cook time: 40 Minutes

Serving: 6

Ingredients

- 4 tablespoons canola oil, divided
- 2 tablespoons lemon juice
- 1-1/2 teaspoons seasoned salt
- 1-1/2 teaspoons dried oregano
- 1-1/2 teaspoons ground cumin
- 1 teaspoon garlic powder
- 1/2 teaspoon chili powder
- 1/2 teaspoon paprika
- 1/2 teaspoon crushed red pepper flakes, optional
- 1-1/2 pounds boneless skinless chicken breasts, cut into thin strips
- 1/2 medium sweet red pepper, julienned
- 1/2 medium green pepper, julienned
- 4 green onions, thinly sliced
- 1/2 cup chopped onion
- 6 flour tortillas (8 inches), warmed

- Optional: Shredded cheddar cheese, taco sauce, salsa, guacamole, sliced red onions and sour cream

Instructions

1. In a large bowl, combine 2 tablespoons oil, lemon juice and seasonings; add the chicken. Turn to coat; cover. Refrigerate for 1-4 hours. , In a large cast-iron or other heavy skillet, saute peppers and onions in remaining oil until crisp-tender. Remove and keep warm. , Drain chicken, discarding marinade. In the same skillet, cook chicken over medium-high heat until no longer pink, 5-6 minutes. Return pepper mixture to pan; heat through. , Spoon filling down the center of tortillas; fold in half. Serve with toppings as desired.

Prep Time: 35 Minutes

Cook Time: 45 Minutes

Servings: 3

Ingredients

- 2 cans (28 ounces each) diced tomatoes, undrained
- 1 can (12 ounces) tomato paste
- 1-1/2 cups water, divided
- 3 tablespoons grated onion
- 1 tablespoon sugar
- 1-1/2 teaspoons dried oregano
- 1 bay leaf
- 1-1/4 teaspoons salt, divided
- 1 teaspoon minced garlic, divided
- 3/4 teaspoon pepper, divided
- 6 slices day-old bread, torn into pieces
- 2 large eggs, lightly beaten
- 1/2 cup grated Parmesan cheese
- 2 tablespoons minced fresh parsley
- 1 pound ground beef
- Hot cooked spaghetti

- Additional Parmesan cheese, optional

Instructions

1. In a Dutch oven, combine the tomatoes, tomato paste, 1 cup water, onion, sugar, oregano, bay leaf and 1/2 teaspoon each of salt, garlic and pepper. Bring to a boil. Reduce heat and simmer, uncovered, for 1-1/4 hours., Meanwhile, soak bread in remaining water. Squeeze out excess moisture. In a large bowl, combine the bread, eggs, Parmesan cheese, parsley and remaining salt, garlic and pepper. Crumble beef over mixture and mix well. Shape into thirty-six 1-1/2-in. meatballs. , Preheat oven to 400°. Place meatballs on a rack in a shallow baking pan. Bake, uncovered, until no longer pink, 20 minutes; drain. Transfer to spaghetti sauce. Simmer, uncovered, until heated through, stirring occasionally. Discard bay leaf. Serve with spaghetti; if desired, top with additional Parmesan.

Prep Time: 35 Minutes

Cook Time: 45 Minutes

Servings: 3

Ingredients

- 2 tablespoons olive oil
- 3 whole garlic cloves, peeled
- 2 pig's feet
- 1 pound pork neck bones
- 2 (6 ounce) cans tomato paste
- 1 ½ cups water
- 2 (28 ounce) cans tomato puree
- 1 tablespoon white sugar
- 1 teaspoon black pepper
- ¾ teaspoon baking soda
- 1 (16 ounce) loaf fresh Italian bread, torn into 2-inch pieces
- 1 cup water
- 6 eggs, beaten
- 1 pound ground pork
- 1 pound ground veal

- 1 pound ground beef

- 1 tablespoon olive oil

- 1 clove garlic, minced

- 2 tablespoons chopped fresh basil

- salt and pepper to taste

- 6 hard-boiled eggs, peeled

Instructions

2. Heat 2 tablespoons of olive oil over medium heat in the bottom of a large saucepan, and fry the garlic cloves 5 to 8 minutes, until brown and fragrant. Remove the garlic cloves and set aside. Place the pig's feet and pork neck bones in the saucepan and fry, turning occasionally, until the meat and bones have browned, about 15 minutes.

3. Return the garlic cloves to the saucepan, and stir in the tomato paste and 1 1/2 cups of water. Bring to a boil, and pour in the tomato puree. Reduce heat to low, and simmer for about 3 hours, stirring from the bottom often to prevent burning, until the pig's feet are tender and the mixture begins to thicken. Stir in the sugar, pepper, and baking soda. Continue to simmer while you prepare the meatballs.

4. Soak the torn bread with 1 cup of water in a bowl. Squeeze excess water out of the bread, and place the bread in a large bowl with the 6 beaten eggs, ground pork, ground veal, and ground beef. Mix thoroughly and form into 24 meatballs about 2 1/2 inches in diameter.

5. Heat 1 tablespoon olive oil in a large skillet over medium heat, stir in the minced garlic and chopped fresh basil, let them cook for about 1 minute, and then add the meatballs. Season with salt and pepper to taste, and fry them on all sides until brown, about 15 minutes, working in batches, if necessary.

6. Place the browned meatballs, along with the oil, garlic, and basil from the skillet into the sauce, stirring lightly to avoid breaking them. Add the whole hard-boiled eggs, and simmer for about 1 1/2 more hours, until the meatballs are cooked, the sauce is thick, and all the flavors have blended.

25. Kittencal's Italian Tomato Pasta Sauce and Parmesan Meatballs

Prep Time: 40 Minutes

Cook Time: 55 Minutes

Servings: 3

Ingredients

- prepared meatballs, Italian Melt-In-Your-Mouth Meatballs)
- olive oil (to cover bottom of the pot)
- 1 large onion, chopped
- 6 large garlic cloves, finely chopped (or to taste)
- 1 -2 bay leaf
- 1 tablespoon dried oregano (rubbed with fingers to release the oils)
- 1 tablespoon dried basil (rubbed with fingers to release the oils)
- 1 -2 tablespoon salt (or to taste)
- 1 teaspoon fresh ground black pepper (or to taste)
- 1 teaspoon crushed red pepper flakes (optional or to taste)
- 1 (6 ounce) can tomato paste

- 1/3-1/2 cup dry red wine (or to taste)
- 2 (28 ounce) cans crushed tomatoes (can use 3 cans if you plan of freezing some sauce)
- 2 (28 ounce) cans diced tomatoes, well drained
- 1 tablespoon sugar (optional and to be added in the last 30 minutes of cooking time)

Instructions

1. Prepare the meatball recipe as directed on the recipe; transfer to a plate cover with plastic wrap and refrigerate until ready to use (the meatballs may be prepared up to 1 day in advance).
2. Drain the diced tomatoes over a strainer.
3. Coat bottom of large heavy-bottomed pot with olive oil, heat over medium heat.
4. Saute onion with bay leaf, oregano, basil, salt, black pepper and crushed chili peppers for about 5-7 minutes or until the onions are transparent.
5. Add in fresh garlic; cook stirring for 2 minutes.
6. Add the tomato paste;mix and stir for about 2 minutes or until well combined with the onion mixture.
7. Add in the wine; stir well to combine.

8. Add the 2 cans crushed tomatoes (can use 3 cans if you are freezing some sauce) and the drained diced tomatoes, stir and bring to a light boil; boil for 5-8 minutes then reduce heat to low.

9. Add in uncooked meatballs to the sauce (if you are adding the meatballs uncooked do not stir for 30 minutes or you may run the risk of them falling apart in the simmering sauce).

10. Simmer uncovered on low heat for about 3-5 hours (the longer you simmer uncovered the thicker and richer your sauce will be so don't be afraid to simmer even 6 hours!) adding more salt if desired.

11. Skim off any fat that might gather on top of sauce.

12. Allow to cool to room temperature then refrigerate (with the meatballs in the sauce) a minimum of 1 day or up to 4 days before using.

13. Use as much as desired then freeze the rest for another meal, just reheat the sauce on top of the stove or heat in microwave (this will freeze well for up to 6 months).

14. Note: if desired, you can bake the meatballs in the oven before adding to the sauce.

Prep Time: 15 Minutes

Cook Time: 50 Minutes

Servings: 3

Ingredients

- 1 lb fresh spinach (washed and dried)
- 4 large fresh white button mushrooms (thinly sliced)
- 1/4 cup crumbled cooked bacon
- 1 small red onion, thinly sliced (optional)
- 1/4 cup crumbled blue cheese (or use feta cheese or Parmesan)
- 1 1/2 cups croutons (or 1/4 cup toasted sunflower Garlic Croutons
- black pepper
- salt (optional)
- 3 hard-cooked hard-boiled eggs (peeled sliced into wedges)
- 1 teaspoon fresh minced garlic
- 1 teaspoon salt (or to taste)
- 3 teaspoons Dijon mustard
- 3 -4 teaspoons honey (or to taste)

- 6 tablespoons balsamic vinegar
- 1/2 cup olive oil, plus
- 2 tablespoons olive oil
- black pepper

Instructions

1. For the dressing; in a bowl whisk together garlic, salt, Dijon, honey and balsamic vinegar; add in olive oil in a slow steady stream until emulsified.
2. Adjust honey amount adding in more if desired for a sweeter taste, then season with more salt if needed, and black pepper.
3. Chill for a minimum of 2 hours before using.
4. For salad; place the spinach leaves in a large glass bowl; top with sliced mushrooms, bacon, blue cheese or feta cheese, croutons and sliced red onion (if using).
5. Toss all ingredients together with salad forks.
6. Season with black pepper (and salt if desired).
7. Place the egg wedges all around inside edges of bowl.
8. Serve with prepared dressing on the side.

Prep Time: 25 Minutes

Cook Time: 40 Minutes

Servings: 6

Ingredients

- 1 French baguette, stale, cut into 1/2 inch cubes
- 1/3 cup butter, I used Smart Balance
- 1/3 cup olive oil
- 1/2 teaspoon dried oregano
- 1/2 teaspoon dried basil
- 1/2 teaspoon dried thyme
- 1/2 teaspoon dried tarragon
- 1/2 teaspoon salt (or to taste)
- 1 teaspoon course ground pepper
- 1 teaspoon course granulated garlic

Instructions

1. Preheat oven to 200.
2. Place cubed bread in big mixing bowl.

3. Melt butter in small sauce pan. Add olive oil, stir, remove from heat.

4. Add in all the spices, salt and pepper.

5. Drizzle half over bread, toss to coat. Add second half to desired amout of flavor(for stronger flavor add all, for light flavor only use half), toss again to coat well.

6. Spread evenly in single layer on an ungreased cookie sheet.

7. Bake for a about 2 hours to get all the moisture out.

8. Turn oven up to 300 let cook for 15 minute and mix them up and cook for about 15 min longer or until nice and toasted. Cool on paper towel then store in an airtight container.

Prep Time: 15 Minutes

Cook Time: 30 Minutes

Servings: 6

Ingredients

- 2 cups ketchup
- 2 cups tomato sauce
- 1 1/4 cups brown sugar
- 1 1/4 cups red wine vinegar
- 1/2 cup unsulphured molasses
- 4 teaspoons hickory-flavored liquid smoke
- 2 tablespoons butter
- 1/2 teaspoon garlic powder
- 1/2 teaspoon onion powder
- 1/4 teaspoon chili powder
- 1 teaspoon paprika
- 1/2 teaspoon celery seed
- 1/4 teaspoon ground cinnamon
- 1/2 teaspoon cayenne pepper
- 1 teaspoon salt
- 1 teaspoon fresh coarse ground black pepper

Instructions

1. In a large saucepan over medium heat, mix together the ketchup, tomato sauce, brown sugar, wine vinegar, molasses, liquid smoke and butter. Season with garlic powder, onion powder, chili powder, paprika, celery seed, cinnamon, cayenne, salt and pepper.

2. Reduce heat to low, and simmer for up to 20 minutes. For thicker sauce, simmer longer, and for thinner, less time is needed. Sauce can also be thinned using a bit of water if necessary. Brush sauce onto any kind of meat during the last 10 minutes of cooking.

3. My Note: It's thick, sweet and spicy and beautiful in color! To try it out. first I cut the servings to 12. I followed the scaled measurements except only used a pinch of cayenne and chili powder. Concern was it may be too spicy for kids. I did not have celery seed, so I had to leave it out. If you like a sweet and spicy sauce you must try this recipe. I will use this on chicken, pulled pork and ribs. UPDATE: I've made this again using the celery seed and think I like the taste without it. Also for a nice thick sauce it is necessary to simmer on low for at least 20 minutes. And advice to anyone wanting to make it, don't leave out the liquid smoke! I didn't have any, so I was just

going to leave it out, but then my son offered to buy me some and when we added it it was SO much better and really added to the flavor. Only suggestions are that oil can be substituted for the butter or left out alltogether, the molasses can be reduced and it's still sweet, and the chili powder, cayenne, and pepper should probably be doubled. Red pepper is also wonderful for the flavor.

4. I am helping in catering a wedding reception the end of this month and needed a sauce I could call my own, so my kitchen was tore up from the floor up! I measured the spices and saved them for later, then I mixed up the liquids over a slow flame, I did not have any red wine vinegar, but I did have some marsala I mixed 1/4c. and the balance I used of white vinegar, I did not add the butter, I figured the fat from the meat would be enough and I wanted it to have some table time. The sauce tasted good but it had no depth, I only used 3 teaspoons of liquid smoke, and let it simmer for a while. Once I added the spices it was the bomb! This is the best sauce I have ever tasted. The spices are fantastic! Whoever thought cinnamon would work in a bbq sauce? I told my husband, we have to go get a piece of meat to go with the sauce. Thanks for sharing,

this is great! I also simmered it for about 1 1/2 hours to thicken, Uuummm finger licken good! I will serve it with pulled pork and baked chicken, I am sure you could serve this with fingernails, and toe-jams.

5. I made just as is (but halved the recipe= 1 1/2 C) and I simmered it for about 50 minutes. The next day it was nice and thick. The liquid smoke is a great flavor in this (a must!), and mellows out by the next day. I also used a pinch of cayenne, so the kids could eat it. I used this on some pulled pork, next it'll go on grilled chicken. Next time I'll make the full batch to keep on hand.

6.

Prep Time: 35 Minutes

Cook Time: 50 Minutes

Servings: 4

Ingredients

- ⅓ cup soy sauce
- ½ cup olive oil
- ⅓ cup fresh lemon juice
- ¼ cup Worcestershire sauce
- 1 ½ tablespoons garlic powder
- 3 tablespoons dried basil
- 1 ½ tablespoons dried parsley flakes
- 1 teaspoon ground white pepper
- ¼ teaspoon hot pepper sauce
- 1 teaspoon dried minced garli

Instructions

1. Place the soy sauce, olive oil, lemon juice, Worcestershire sauce, garlic powder, basil, parsley,

and pepper in a blender. Add hot pepper sauce and garlic, if desired. Blend on high speed for 30 seconds until thoroughly mixed.

2. Pour marinade over desired type of meat. Cover, and refrigerate for up to 8 hours. Cook meat as desired.

Prep Time: 45 Minutes

Cook Time: 55 Minutes

Servings: 4

Ingredients

- 5 oz baby spinach
- 1 cup strawberry, sliced
- ½ cup blueberry
- ½ red onion, thinly sliced
- 1 sweet apple, cored, halved and thinly sliced
- 1 cup candied walnuts, chopped
- 1 cup strawberry
- ¼ cup balsamic vinegar
- ¼ cup extra virgin olive oil
- 1 tablespoon dijon mustard
- 1 tablespoon honey
- 1 clove garlic, minced
- ¼ teaspoon salt
- ¼ teaspoon pepper

- ⅔ cup feta cheese, as desired

Instructions

4. For the dressing, push a straw through the strawberries from the tip to the green top to remove the hull. (Or you can cut it off with a knife!)
5. Add the rest of the dressing ingredients.
6. Blend until smooth. Refrigerate.
7. Cut strawberries, apple, and onion into slices.
8. Combine all the salad ingredients in a large bowl.
9. Drizzle with desired amount of dressing and toss to coat. (Spinach wilts easily, don't add dressing until ready to eat!)
10. Sprinkle feta cheese on top and serve.
11. Enjoy!

www.ingramcontent.com/pod-product-compliance
Lightning Source LLC
Chambersburg PA
CBHW051839250726
48659CB00005B/1933